You Have Got This.

What Are You Aiming For?

This may seem like a blindingly obvious question but…
Why are you bothering with this rehab at all?

'Because the doctor said so' isn't good enough, neither is 'I want to get back to full strength'. Neither of those will keep you going through the tough times. Take some time to drill down into this and figure out exactly what it is that you are aiming for and what will really motivate you to stick with it.

Do you miss...
- Leaping over the stream on your morning run?
- Standing on the pedals as you blast round the final corner of the trail?
- The smell of chalk in the air at the gym?
- The camaraderie of figuring out a boulder problem together?
- Being able to feed yourself lunch?
- The goofy happiness on your dog's face as you take the 'long walk' option?

Whatever the reason is for you, write it down in as much detail as you can. You have to know what the end goal is, and remind yourself of why it is worth aiming for. The journey ahead can be tough, knowing why you are persisting, and what success looks like, is important to keep you motivated.

You are looking for a goal that puts a rocket under you, lights you up like a massive sparkler or makes you grin like a happy loon anticipating being able to do it again.

What am I aiming for?

What exactly will success look like?

Overcoming The Obstacles

Or, "What Will I Do When It Doesn't Go To Plan?"
(This Is Absolutely Essential, DO NOT Skip This Step!)

There will always be obstacles and things that get in the way of doing your rehab exercises, maybe just on certain days or every single day. These can easily derail you and make you feel like you 'can't' do your exercises, or that there isn't any point even trying because you never seem to do them 'properly' if at all. The solution to this is figuring out how to get around the obstacles before they even pop up in front of you.

When you are tired and have to make a decision (for instance, "Do I do my exercises or just go straight to bed because I'm tired?") your brain panics and generally steers you to take the option with the most immediate short-term gratification. This is fine occasionally, but when it happens regularly then you are stuck making absolutely no progress towards your longer term goal (the one that you really truly care about and lights you up like a fizzy firework, remember?).

The way to get out of this depressing loop (feeling guilty about not progressing but never actually moving forward) is to decide in advance what your options are in these scenarios and how you will handle them. This means that your brain doesn't have to do any tough decision-making, it just says "oh yes, when this comes up we do this...". This takes away the panic and stress of having to make a choice, you already know how to deal with this obstacle so you just set that solution into motion.

So "Do I do my exercises or just go straight to bed because I am tired?" becomes easy to answer with "I do a half set of each of my exercises and an extra half set in the morning", because this is what you had already decided.

Take the time to think about what generally crops up and stops your good intentions in their tracks. Figure out when you can fit your exercises in even if you don't manage them when you planned to.
Solve as many obstacles as you can and get your back-up plans in place to help you out if life throws you one of those curveballs that it loves to do!. It is honestly way easier to figure out the solution now and save yourself future stress.

'What If I Completely Fall Off The Wagon?'
Yes there will still be times when even this doesn't work and you don't do your exercises that day, or that week. Maybe you fall right off the wagon and just lie there on the track. Don't waste time worrying about what has been or what you haven't done, you can't change that.

Just focus on what you can do TODAY and figure out how you can make it work right now, even just a little bit.
Don't even worry about tomorrow, just do it today. You can figure out tomorrow when it comes.

A sneaky trick is also to tell yourself that you will give yourself a day off TOMORROW, but today you do the exercises. Generally by the time tomorrow comes you will be in a different place and just get on and do them, or you can pull the same trick!

Potential Obstacles	Solutions

Potential Obstacles	Solutions

Using The Tracker Pages

Honestly, do what you like with them. It's your book, rock on with your bad self and unleash your style in whichever way feels best to you. Just make sure you do!
Our brains are wired to get a kick of satisfaction from checking things off (success, win, triumph, conquer, done, woohoo!), which is why trackers like this work so well.

There is space for the date and any other notes for the day at the top, and slots for 10 exercises. Most injury rehab programs won't give you more than this as it starts to get overwhelming. If you have more than 10 then pick the key ones or get a second tracker book!

Exercise 10:
Notes:

Tip: Name your exercise (I love assigning silly names, like arm monster walk or chin cha-cha, anything to keep me smiling!). Boxes are in threes for easy counting and can be coloured, filled with reps, checked, ignored because you wrote notes instead, whatever works for you!

Today:

This is a space for any additional notes on the day... Did you get an extra 2 degrees of movement? Was it easier after an ice swim? Did you find a really inspiring story? Did you have a physio appointment? Did you find a new rehab soundtrack?

Starting Strong.

Will Finish Stronger.

Date:

Exercise 1:
Notes:

Exercise 2:
Notes:

Exercise 3:
Notes:

Exercise 4:
Notes:

Exercise 5:
Notes:

Exercise 6:
Notes:

Exercise 7:
Notes:

Exercise 8:
Notes:

Exercise 9:
Notes:

Exercise 10:
Notes:

Today:

Date:

Exercise 1:
Notes:

Exercise 2:
Notes:

Exercise 3:
Notes:

Exercise 4:
Notes:

Exercise 5:
Notes:

Exercise 6:
Notes:

Exercise 7:
Notes:

Exercise 8:
Notes:

Exercise 9:
Notes:

Exercise 10:
Notes:

Today:

Date:

Exercise 1:
Notes:

Exercise 2:
Notes:

Exercise 3:
Notes:

Exercise 4:
Notes:

Exercise 5:
Notes:

Exercise 6:
Notes:

Exercise 7:
Notes:

Exercise 8:
Notes:

Exercise 9:
Notes:

Exercise 10:
Notes:

Today:

Date:

Exercise 1:
Notes:

Exercise 2:
Notes:

Exercise 3:
Notes:

Exercise 4:
Notes:

Exercise 5:
Notes:

Exercise 6:
Notes:

Exercise 7:
Notes:

Exercise 8:
Notes:

Exercise 9:
Notes:

Exercise 10:
Notes:

Today:

Date:

Exercise 1:
Notes:

Exercise 2:
Notes:

Exercise 3:
Notes:

Exercise 4:
Notes:

Exercise 5:
Notes:

Exercise 6:
Notes:

Exercise 7:
Notes:

Exercise 8:
Notes:

Exercise 9:
Notes:

Exercise 10:
Notes:

Today:

Date:

Exercise 1:
Notes:

Exercise 2:
Notes:

Exercise 3:
Notes:

Exercise 4:
Notes:

Exercise 5:
Notes:

Exercise 6:
Notes:

Exercise 7:
Notes:

Exercise 8:
Notes:

Exercise 9:
Notes:

Exercise 10:
Notes:

Today:

Date:

Exercise 1:
Notes:

Exercise 2:
Notes:

Exercise 3:
Notes:

Exercise 4:
Notes:

Exercise 5:
Notes:

Exercise 6:
Notes:

Exercise 7:
Notes:

Exercise 8:
Notes:

Exercise 9:
Notes:

Exercise 10:
Notes:

Today:

Date:

Exercise 1:
Notes:

Exercise 2:
Notes:

Exercise 3:
Notes:

Exercise 4:
Notes:

Exercise 5:
Notes:

Exercise 6:
Notes:

Exercise 7:
Notes:

Exercise 8:
Notes:

Exercise 9:
Notes:

Exercise 10:
Notes:

Today:

Date:

Exercise 1:
Notes:

Exercise 2:
Notes:

Exercise 3:
Notes:

Exercise 4:
Notes:

Exercise 5:
Notes:

Exercise 6:
Notes:

Exercise 7:
Notes:

Exercise 8:
Notes:

Exercise 9:
Notes:

Exercise 10:
Notes:

Today:

Date:

Exercise 1:
Notes:

Exercise 2:
Notes:

Exercise 3:
Notes:

Exercise 4:
Notes:

Exercise 5:
Notes:

Exercise 6:
Notes:

Exercise 7:
Notes:

Exercise 8:
Notes:

Exercise 9:
Notes:

Exercise 10:
Notes:

Today:

Do Something Today That Your Future Self Will Thank You For

Check In Time...

So, what's working well?

Is there anything I need to change up?

What inspired me recently?

Date:

Exercise 1:
Notes:

Exercise 2:
Notes:

Exercise 3:
Notes:

Exercise 4:
Notes:

Exercise 5:
Notes:

Exercise 6:
Notes:

Exercise 7:
Notes:

Exercise 8:
Notes:

Exercise 9:
Notes:

Exercise 10:
Notes:

Today:

Date:

Exercise 1:
Notes:

Exercise 2:
Notes:

Exercise 3:
Notes:

Exercise 4:
Notes:

Exercise 5:
Notes:

Exercise 6:
Notes:

Exercise 7:
Notes:

Exercise 8:
Notes:

Exercise 9:
Notes:

Exercise 10:
Notes:

Today:

Date:

Exercise 1:
Notes:

Exercise 2:
Notes:

Exercise 3:
Notes:

Exercise 4:
Notes:

Exercise 5:
Notes:

Exercise 6:
Notes:

Exercise 7:
Notes:

Exercise 8:
Notes:

Exercise 9:
Notes:

Exercise 10:
Notes:

Today:

Date:

Exercise 1:
Notes:

Exercise 2:
Notes:

Exercise 3:
Notes:

Exercise 4:
Notes:

Exercise 5:
Notes:

Exercise 6:
Notes:

Exercise 7:
Notes:

Exercise 8:
Notes:

Exercise 9:
Notes:

Exercise 10:
Notes:

Today:

Date:

Exercise 1:
Notes:

Exercise 2:
Notes:

Exercise 3:
Notes:

Exercise 4:
Notes:

Exercise 5:
Notes:

Exercise 6:
Notes:

Exercise 7:
Notes:

Exercise 8:
Notes:

Exercise 9:
Notes:

Exercise 10:
Notes:

Today:

Date:

Exercise 1:
Notes:

Exercise 2:
Notes:

Exercise 3:
Notes:

Exercise 4:
Notes:

Exercise 5:
Notes:

Exercise 6:
Notes:

Exercise 7:
Notes:

Exercise 8:
Notes:

Exercise 9:
Notes:

Exercise 10:
Notes:

Today:

You Rock!

YES, YOU DO!

NEVER DOUBT IT.

Date:

Exercise 1:
Notes:

Exercise 2:
Notes:

Exercise 3:
Notes:

Exercise 4:
Notes:

Exercise 5:
Notes:

Exercise 6:
Notes:

Exercise 7:
Notes:

Exercise 8:
Notes:

Exercise 9:
Notes:

Exercise 10:
Notes:

Today:

Date:

Exercise 1:
Notes:

Exercise 2:
Notes:

Exercise 3:
Notes:

Exercise 4:
Notes:

Exercise 5:
Notes:

Exercise 6:
Notes:

Exercise 7:
Notes:

Exercise 8:
Notes:

Exercise 9:
Notes:

Exercise 10:
Notes:

Today:

Date:

Exercise 1:
Notes:

Exercise 2:
Notes:

Exercise 3:
Notes:

Exercise 4:
Notes:

Exercise 5:
Notes:

Exercise 6:
Notes:

Exercise 7:
Notes:

Exercise 8:
Notes:

Exercise 9:
Notes:

Exercise 10:
Notes:

Today:

Date:

Exercise 1:
Notes:

Exercise 2:
Notes:

Exercise 3:
Notes:

Exercise 4:
Notes:

Exercise 5:
Notes:

Exercise 6:
Notes:

Exercise 7:
Notes:

Exercise 8:
Notes:

Exercise 9:
Notes:

Exercise 10:
Notes:

Today:

Date:

Exercise 1:
Notes:

Exercise 2:
Notes:

Exercise 3:
Notes:

Exercise 4:
Notes:

Exercise 5:
Notes:

Exercise 6:
Notes:

Exercise 7:
Notes:

Exercise 8:
Notes:

Exercise 9:
Notes:

Exercise 10:
Notes:

Today:

Date:

Exercise 1:
Notes:

Exercise 2:
Notes:

Exercise 3:
Notes:

Exercise 4:
Notes:

Exercise 5:
Notes:

Exercise 6:
Notes:

Exercise 7:
Notes:

Exercise 8:
Notes:

Exercise 9:
Notes:

Exercise 10:
Notes:

Today:

Date:

Exercise 1:
Notes:

Exercise 2:
Notes:

Exercise 3:
Notes:

Exercise 4:
Notes:

Exercise 5:
Notes:

Exercise 6:
Notes:

Exercise 7:
Notes:

Exercise 8:
Notes:

Exercise 9:
Notes:

Exercise 10:
Notes:

Today:

Date:

Exercise 1:
Notes:

Exercise 2:
Notes:

Exercise 3:
Notes:

Exercise 4:
Notes:

Exercise 5:
Notes:

Exercise 6:
Notes:

Exercise 7:
Notes:

Exercise 8:
Notes:

Exercise 9:
Notes:

Exercise 10:
Notes:

Today:

Date:

Exercise 1:
Notes:

Exercise 2:
Notes:

Exercise 3:
Notes:

Exercise 4:
Notes:

Exercise 5:
Notes:

Exercise 6:
Notes:

Exercise 7:
Notes:

Exercise 8:
Notes:

Exercise 9:
Notes:

Exercise 10:
Notes:

Today:

Date:

Exercise 1:
Notes:

Exercise 2:
Notes:

Exercise 3:
Notes:

Exercise 4:
Notes:

Exercise 5:
Notes:

Exercise 6:
Notes:

Exercise 7:
Notes:

Exercise 8:
Notes:

Exercise 9:
Notes:

Exercise 10:
Notes:

Today:

Take Your Time.
Do It Right.
Recover Strong.

Check In Time...

Has my end goal changed at all?

Any new obstacles I need to figure out
a solution to?

Date:

Exercise 1:
Notes:

Exercise 2:
Notes:

Exercise 3:
Notes:

Exercise 4:
Notes:

Exercise 5:
Notes:

Exercise 6:
Notes:

Exercise 7:
Notes:

Exercise 8:
Notes:

Exercise 9:
Notes:

Exercise 10:
Notes:

Today:

Date:

Exercise 1:
Notes:

Exercise 2:
Notes:

Exercise 3:
Notes:

Exercise 4:
Notes:

Exercise 5:
Notes:

Exercise 6:
Notes:

Exercise 7:
Notes:

Exercise 8:
Notes:

Exercise 9:
Notes:

Exercise 10:
Notes:

Today:

Date:

Exercise 1:
Notes:

Exercise 2:
Notes:

Exercise 3:
Notes:

Exercise 4:
Notes:

Exercise 5:
Notes:

Exercise 6:
Notes:

Exercise 7:
Notes:

Exercise 8:
Notes:

Exercise 9:
Notes:

Exercise 10:
Notes:

Today:

Date:

Exercise 1:
Notes:

Exercise 2:
Notes:

Exercise 3:
Notes:

Exercise 4:
Notes:

Exercise 5:
Notes:

Exercise 6:
Notes:

Exercise 7:
Notes:

Exercise 8:
Notes:

Exercise 9:
Notes:

Exercise 10:
Notes:

Today:

Date:

Exercise 1:
Notes:

Exercise 2:
Notes:

Exercise 3:
Notes:

Exercise 4:
Notes:

Exercise 5:
Notes:

Exercise 6:
Notes:

Exercise 7:
Notes:

Exercise 8:
Notes:

Exercise 9:
Notes:

Exercise 10:
Notes:

Today:

Date:

Exercise 1:
Notes:

Exercise 2:
Notes:

Exercise 3:
Notes:

Exercise 4:
Notes:

Exercise 5:
Notes:

Exercise 6:
Notes:

Exercise 7:
Notes:

Exercise 8:
Notes:

Exercise 9:
Notes:

Exercise 10:
Notes:

Today:

This is to certify that I

Am freaking awesome and have got this. Go me!

Check In Time...

So, what's working well?

Is there anything I need to change up?

What inspired me recently?

Date:

Exercise 1:
Notes:

Exercise 2:
Notes:

Exercise 3:
Notes:

Exercise 4:
Notes:

Exercise 5:
Notes:

Exercise 6:
Notes:

Exercise 7:
Notes:

Exercise 8:
Notes:

Exercise 9:
Notes:

Exercise 10:
Notes:

Today:

Date:

Exercise 1:
Notes:

Exercise 2:
Notes:

Exercise 3:
Notes:

Exercise 4:
Notes:

Exercise 5:
Notes:

Exercise 6:
Notes:

Exercise 7:
Notes:

Exercise 8:
Notes:

Exercise 9:
Notes:

Exercise 10:
Notes:

Today:

Date:

Exercise 1:
Notes:

Exercise 2:
Notes:

Exercise 3:
Notes:

Exercise 4:
Notes:

Exercise 5:
Notes:

Exercise 6:
Notes:

Exercise 7:
Notes:

Exercise 8:
Notes:

Exercise 9:
Notes:

Exercise 10:
Notes:

Today:

Date:

Exercise 1:
Notes:

Exercise 2:
Notes:

Exercise 3:
Notes:

Exercise 4:
Notes:

Exercise 5:
Notes:

Exercise 6:
Notes:

Exercise 7:
Notes:

Exercise 8:
Notes:

Exercise 9:
Notes:

Exercise 10:
Notes:

Today:

Date:

Exercise 1:
Notes:

Exercise 2:
Notes:

Exercise 3:
Notes:

Exercise 4:
Notes:

Exercise 5:
Notes:

Exercise 6:
Notes:

Exercise 7:
Notes:

Exercise 8:
Notes:

Exercise 9:
Notes:

Exercise 10:
Notes:

Today:

Date:

Exercise 1:
Notes:

Exercise 2:
Notes:

Exercise 3:
Notes:

Exercise 4:
Notes:

Exercise 5:
Notes:

Exercise 6:
Notes:

Exercise 7:
Notes:

Exercise 8:
Notes:

Exercise 9:
Notes:

Exercise 10:
Notes:

Today:

Date:

Exercise 1:
Notes:

Exercise 2:
Notes:

Exercise 3:
Notes:

Exercise 4:
Notes:

Exercise 5:
Notes:

Exercise 6:
Notes:

Exercise 7:
Notes:

Exercise 8:
Notes:

Exercise 9:
Notes:

Exercise 10:
Notes:

Today:

Date:

Exercise 1:
Notes:

Exercise 2:
Notes:

Exercise 3:
Notes:

Exercise 4:
Notes:

Exercise 5:
Notes:

Exercise 6:
Notes:

Exercise 7:
Notes:

Exercise 8:
Notes:

Exercise 9:
Notes:

Exercise 10:
Notes:

Today:

Date:

Exercise 1:
Notes:

Exercise 2:
Notes:

Exercise 3:
Notes:

Exercise 4:
Notes:

Exercise 5:
Notes:

Exercise 6:
Notes:

Exercise 7:
Notes:

Exercise 8:
Notes:

Exercise 9:
Notes:

Exercise 10:
Notes:

Today:

Date:

Exercise 1:
Notes:

Exercise 2:
Notes:

Exercise 3:
Notes:

Exercise 4:
Notes:

Exercise 5:
Notes:

Exercise 6:
Notes:

Exercise 7:
Notes:

Exercise 8:
Notes:

Exercise 9:
Notes:

Exercise 10:
Notes:

Today:

Check In Time...

Has my end goal changed at all?

Any new obstacles I need to figure out
a solution to?

Future You Says "Thank You" For Sticking With It!

Date:

Exercise 1:
Notes:

Exercise 2:
Notes:

Exercise 3:
Notes:

Exercise 4:
Notes:

Exercise 5:
Notes:

Exercise 6:
Notes:

Exercise 7:
Notes:

Exercise 8:
Notes:

Exercise 9:
Notes:

Exercise 10:
Notes:

Today:

Date:

Exercise 1:
Notes:

Exercise 2:
Notes:

Exercise 3:
Notes:

Exercise 4:
Notes:

Exercise 5:
Notes:

Exercise 6:
Notes:

Exercise 7:
Notes:

Exercise 8:
Notes:

Exercise 9:
Notes:

Exercise 10:
Notes:

Today:

Date:

Exercise 1:
Notes:

Exercise 2:
Notes:

Exercise 3:
Notes:

Exercise 4:
Notes:

Exercise 5:
Notes:

Exercise 6:
Notes:

Exercise 7:
Notes:

Exercise 8:
Notes:

Exercise 9:
Notes:

Exercise 10:
Notes:

Today:

Date:

Exercise 1:
Notes:

Exercise 2:
Notes:

Exercise 3:
Notes:

Exercise 4:
Notes:

Exercise 5:
Notes:

Exercise 6:
Notes:

Exercise 7:
Notes:

Exercise 8:
Notes:

Exercise 9:
Notes:

Exercise 10:
Notes:

Today:

Date:

Exercise 1:
Notes:

Exercise 2:
Notes:

Exercise 3:
Notes:

Exercise 4:
Notes:

Exercise 5:
Notes:

Exercise 6:
Notes:

Exercise 7:
Notes:

Exercise 8:
Notes:

Exercise 9:
Notes:

Exercise 10:
Notes:

Today:

Date:

Exercise 1:
Notes:

Exercise 2:
Notes:

Exercise 3:
Notes:

Exercise 4:
Notes:

Exercise 5:
Notes:

Exercise 6:
Notes:

Exercise 7:
Notes:

Exercise 8:
Notes:

Exercise 9:
Notes:

Exercise 10:
Notes:

Today:

Date:

Exercise 1:
Notes:

Exercise 2:
Notes:

Exercise 3:
Notes:

Exercise 4:
Notes:

Exercise 5:
Notes:

Exercise 6:
Notes:

Exercise 7:
Notes:

Exercise 8:
Notes:

Exercise 9:
Notes:

Exercise 10:
Notes:

Today:

Date:

Exercise 1:
Notes:

Exercise 2:
Notes:

Exercise 3:
Notes:

Exercise 4:
Notes:

Exercise 5:
Notes:

Exercise 6:
Notes:

Exercise 7:
Notes:

Exercise 8:
Notes:

Exercise 9:
Notes:

Exercise 10:
Notes:

Today:

Date:

Exercise 1:
Notes:

Exercise 2:
Notes:

Exercise 3:
Notes:

Exercise 4:
Notes:

Exercise 5:
Notes:

Exercise 6:
Notes:

Exercise 7:
Notes:

Exercise 8:
Notes:

Exercise 9:
Notes:

Exercise 10:
Notes:

Today:

Date:

Exercise 1:
Notes:

Exercise 2:
Notes:

Exercise 3:
Notes:

Exercise 4:
Notes:

Exercise 5:
Notes:

Exercise 6:
Notes:

Exercise 7:
Notes:

Exercise 8:
Notes:

Exercise 9:
Notes:

Exercise 10:
Notes:

Today:

KEEP GOING!

You Have Got This.

Date:

Exercise 1:
Notes:

Exercise 2:
Notes:

Exercise 3:
Notes:

Exercise 4:
Notes:

Exercise 5:
Notes:

Exercise 6:
Notes:

Exercise 7:
Notes:

Exercise 8:
Notes:

Exercise 9:
Notes:

Exercise 10:
Notes:

Today:

Date:

Exercise 1:
Notes:

Exercise 2:
Notes:

Exercise 3:
Notes:

Exercise 4:
Notes:

Exercise 5:
Notes:

Exercise 6:
Notes:

Exercise 7:
Notes:

Exercise 8:
Notes:

Exercise 9:
Notes:

Exercise 10:
Notes:

Today:

Date:

Exercise 1:
Notes:

Exercise 2:
Notes:

Exercise 3:
Notes:

Exercise 4:
Notes:

Exercise 5:
Notes:

Exercise 6:
Notes:

Exercise 7:
Notes:

Exercise 8:
Notes:

Exercise 9:
Notes:

Exercise 10:
Notes:

Today:

Date:

Exercise 1:
Notes:

Exercise 2:
Notes:

Exercise 3:
Notes:

Exercise 4:
Notes:

Exercise 5:
Notes:

Exercise 6:
Notes:

Exercise 7:
Notes:

Exercise 8:
Notes:

Exercise 9:
Notes:

Exercise 10:
Notes:

Today:

Date:

Exercise 1:
Notes:

Exercise 2:
Notes:

Exercise 3:
Notes:

Exercise 4:
Notes:

Exercise 5:
Notes:

Exercise 6:
Notes:

Exercise 7:
Notes:

Exercise 8:
Notes:

Exercise 9:
Notes:

Exercise 10:
Notes:

Today:

Date:

Exercise 1:
Notes:

Exercise 2:
Notes:

Exercise 3:
Notes:

Exercise 4:
Notes:

Exercise 5:
Notes:

Exercise 6:
Notes:

Exercise 7:
Notes:

Exercise 8:
Notes:

Exercise 9:
Notes:

Exercise 10:
Notes:

Today:

Date:

Exercise 1:
Notes:

Exercise 2:
Notes:

Exercise 3:
Notes:

Exercise 4:
Notes:

Exercise 5:
Notes:

Exercise 6:
Notes:

Exercise 7:
Notes:

Exercise 8:
Notes:

Exercise 9:
Notes:

Exercise 10:
Notes:

Today:

Date:

Exercise 1:
Notes:

Exercise 2:
Notes:

Exercise 3:
Notes:

Exercise 4:
Notes:

Exercise 5:
Notes:

Exercise 6:
Notes:

Exercise 7:
Notes:

Exercise 8:
Notes:

Exercise 9:
Notes:

Exercise 10:
Notes:

Today:

Date:

Exercise 1:
Notes:

Exercise 2:
Notes:

Exercise 3:
Notes:

Exercise 4:
Notes:

Exercise 5:
Notes:

Exercise 6:
Notes:

Exercise 7:
Notes:

Exercise 8:
Notes:

Exercise 9:
Notes:

Exercise 10:
Notes:

Today:

Date:

Exercise 1:
Notes:

Exercise 2:
Notes:

Exercise 3:
Notes:

Exercise 4:
Notes:

Exercise 5:
Notes:

Exercise 6:
Notes:

Exercise 7:
Notes:

Exercise 8:
Notes:

Exercise 9:
Notes:

Exercise 10:
Notes:

Today:

You absolutely deserve a medal

This is way harder than a marathon.